This paper

Dec 12th 2020

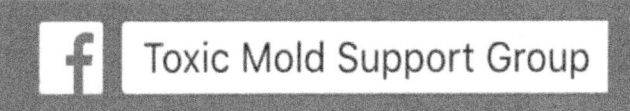

Special thanks to the Toxic Mold Support Group.

I hope you find this information helpful.

Table of Contents

Introduction	7
Disclaimer	11
Chapter 1: What's up with mold?	13
Chapter 2: One in four are susceptible	23
Chapter 3: Ten molds you don't want to find in your home	27
Chapter 4: How to test your home for mold	45
Chapter 5: PPE for mold	57
Chapter 6: Why bleach rarely works but this will	65
Chapter 7: The hidden danger inside your basement — Wooden pallets!	79
Chapter 8: How to Stop Basements Flooding	93

Chapter 9: Outdoor checklist	105
Chapter 10: Indoor checklist	115
Chapter 11: Mold big guns	127
Chapter 12: Hire a pro without getting ripped off	135
Chapter 13: Covered Ground	139
More books by this author	145
Newsletter	147

Copyright 2020 ©

No part of this book is to be copied, republished, or reproduced without written permission from the author. Requests can be made via the James Lilley Facebook page.

You can also stay in my loop through my free newsletter at

writeonjames.com

Write on James.com

Introduction

Hello and thank you for taking the time to open this book. This information will be of interest to those dealing with a mold issue but are unsure why, or how to treat it. Inside, you will learn how to test your home for mold, and how to protect yourself from its toxic effects. We'll also tackle the root causes of mold and how they can impact your health.

This book wastes no time in providing clear, concise answers. Based on my thirty-plus years' experience in construction, I'll tell you how to get the best deal on mold remediation. I will also lift the lid on mold remediation scams.

But first, it's worth noting that microscopic mold spores are all around us. They float into our homes through open windows and can even attach themselves to our clothing and pets. Indeed, it would be quite rare to find a home without any mold spores.

Mold spores are the seeds that help new molds to grow. Like most things in nature, a seed requires nutrients to flourish. Disrupting the supply of food and water is the key to successful mold remediation.

Mold *isn't* too fussy what it eats, cardboard boxes, shoes, carpets, baby clothes, furniture, drywall, and wood will all suffice. Some estimates suggest mold destroys more wood than termites and fires combined!

Fortunately, this book can, and will, help you stop mold in its tracks. The information in this book is easy to read and inexpensive to apply. Without further ado, let's get started!

Disclaimer

This information is intended for information purposes only. While all attempts have been made to verify the content provided in this book, the author does not assume any responsibility for errors, omissions, or alternative interpretations of the issues discussed inside.

The information stated in this book is the sole opinion of James Lilley and should not be taken as expert instructions or commands. Any references to medical conditions should not be taken as medical advice. If you have any type of health issue you must take it up with a qualified health professional. At all times, the reader is one hundred percent responsible for his or her actions.

Adherence to all applicable building laws and regulations is the responsibility of the reader. The author assumes no liability whatsoever for the reader's interpretations on the contents of this book.

Chapter 1: What's up with mold?

Contrary to popular belief, mold has saved countless lives thanks to its contribution as the antibiotic, Penicillin. Mold also plays an important role in breaking down organic materials. It's nature's way of recycling nutrients back into our ecosystem. Without it, life as we know it would cease to exist.

Some of the enzymes found in molds are beneficial to the food industry. For example, mold is used to enhance cheese production. Meanwhile, a species of fungus known as *Aspergillus Tubingensis* was recently found breaking down plastic. This exciting discovery could one day help to save the planet. At this point, you may be asking, how did mold get such a bad reputation?

A little-known fact is that there are over 100,000 different species of mold. Some are relatively harmless; others produce poisonous toxins known as mycotoxins. Mycotoxins are a type of defense mechanism used by mold. Whenever a toxic mold feels threatened, mycotoxins are released into the air. A subtle temperature change could be perceived as a threat. Even a secondary mold competing for growing space could be seen as a threat. Needless to say, molds aren't overly fond of humans that prod and poke them.

Once mycotoxins become airborne, they are small enough to be inhaled. They are large enough to cause a chronic, inflammatory response. Some mycotoxins are considered cytotoxic (toxic to all living cells). This means mycotoxins can have an impact on you *and* your pets.

Other species of mold can spew out aflatoxins which are a class of toxic compounds produced by certain molds. Some aflatoxins can go on to become poisonous carcinogens. You will learn about different mold types later in the book. For now, let's explore how these problematic molds get inside our homes.

Mold reproduces by way of releasing spores into the air. Similar to how a dandelion reseeds itself in the spring. Mold spores are much smaller than dandelion seeds which makes them invisible to the naked eye.

Out in the wild, these tiny mold spores float effortlessly on the wind. Wherever they land, they seek out a source of moisture and begin growing as nature intended. As the mold matures, it is then exposed to sun, rain, and wind. As such, the negative effects of outdoor molds are somewhat diluted.

Indoors, a very different story tends to play out. When mold grows in a bathroom or bedroom, the toxic effects are far more concentrated. Depending on the species of mold, this can create a wide range of health problems. For many, sneezing and wheezing are just the tip of the iceberg.

Microscopic mold spores have no trouble finding their way into your home. They enter through open windows and air-conditioning units. Some get sucked into heating ducts while others can attach themselves to our clothing and pets. It would be highly unusual to find a home *without* mold spores. They are inside my home and I suspect they are also inside yours.

Once inside, mold spores can lay dormant. They have learned to wait for the right opportunity to develop. Mold will thrive in places with insufficient ventilation, a porous material to feed on, and a lick of moisture in the air. This makes attics and basements willing candidates.

Mold also likes to feed on drywall. Drywall is used in the construction industry to build internal walls and ceilings.

Contractors use drywall as it's fast and inexpensive to work with. It's also porous which means it turns to mush when it gets wet. This becomes an ideal surface for mold to snack on.

Alternatives to drywall include brick and breeze blocks. This is how most internal walls are built across Europe. They are then plastered over to give the internal wall a smooth finish. Once painted the two walls look identical. The main difference being that one is prone to mold, the other is not.

In an attempt to combat the moldy drywall problem, fungicides were added to household paints during the 1970's. Unfortunately, this action is now believed to have created mutant strains of mold. Many turned out to be even more potent than the original mold!

Drywall also gives mold a chance to stay out of sight while it gets established. Perhaps being drip-fed by a leaking pipe somewhere inside the wall. By the time it's noticed, the invasive root system of some molds may have spread far and wide. This process can begin happening in as little as 24/48 hours.

To add to the problem, many homeowners believe that spraying bleach on drywall will kill the mold. Sadly, this is unlikely to have any impact. In some cases, it may even cause the mold to spread.

Catching mold early is the key to saving thousands of dollars in remedial costs. As you look around your home pay particular attention to any new watermarks on ceilings. If it's accompanied by a weird, musty smell then it's worthy of further investigation.

Whether you own your home, or you choose to rent it, it pays to be vigilant. Yes, landlords are required by law to provide safe living conditions. This is referred to as "implied warranty of habitability." However, unless you are paying close attention, mold can easily spread from room to room.

By this time, landlords may be unable or unwilling to spend money on mold remediation. Others may cut corners which could make the situation worse. Maybe you have a few thousand dollars to mount a legal battle, and maybe you don't. At all times, remember your health is *your* responsibility.

This brings us back to being aware. Aware of your rights, aware of the health implications, and aware of your options. Personally, if I was dealing with an uncooperative landlord, I'd rather move on and keep my health. I'm not saying giving up your home is easy. But oftentimes, it pays to pick your battles.

If living in a moldy house is making you sick, the chances are you have already lost everything dear to you. The good news is, once you separate yourself from the problem, you'll start to feel much better. *No really, it's true.*

I appreciate moving out isn't an easy option but those caught in a dire mold situation don't have a choice. Walking away is by far the fastest, most effective way to separate yourself from toxic mold. As Oliver Goldsmith once said, *"He who fights and runs away, may live to fight another day."*

Unfortunately, mold spores and mycotoxins are notorious for hitching a free ride. They like to follow you by attaching themselves to your furniture, bedding, and clothes. Just when you thought it couldn't get any worse. Regular laundry detergents are no match for mycotoxins. However, all is not lost. Adding powdered Borax to your wash can help neutralize mold spores. Depending on what kind of mold issue you are dealing with, you may need to kick it up a gear. Applying an additive known as EC3 to the wash can neutralize mycotoxins. EC3 has the power to clean deep without using any harmful chemicals. EC3 also makes an all-natural mold solution. This can be sprayed onto hard surfaces such as wooden furniture and plastics.

If you are in a bind, you can also use white vinegar to help remove some of the mold spores from clothes. Simply fill the washer machine with water, add three cups of white vinegar, and let the clothes sit. After an hour, run the washer machine on its normal cycle. When it comes to drying your clothes, pin them on an outdoor washing line in direct sunshine. This will help to kill any remaining mold spores.

In the next chapter, we'll take a closer look at some of the health problems caused by mold.

Chapter 2: One in four are susceptible

On a cold, blustery day, have you ever noticed how some folks bundle themselves up with a thick winter coat, a woolly hat, and two pairs of gloves? Then there's that other guy, the one trudging through the snow wearing plaid shorts. Here's the thing, we are all wired differently.

By the same token, some people are more susceptible to mold. Estimates suggest that as many as one in four Americans have a genetic predisposition to mold. As we move forward, keep this figure in mind. All too often, a disconnect can occur when only one person in a moldy home gets sick.

If this is you, it's important to be your own health advocate. It's not uncommon for symptoms of mold toxicity to be overlooked by the medical community. It's just not on a busy doctor's radar.

Children and the elderly are particularly susceptible to mold. How sick they become depends on the individual's immune system. Anyone with a weakened immune system will bear the brunt of symptoms. Those fortunate enough to have a robust immune system will fare much better, but still could experience some symptoms.

A lot can also depend on the type of mold. Allergenic molds, as the name suggests, provoke an allergic reaction. This can result in itchy, watery eyes, a runny nose, a sore throat, a dry cough, headaches, skin rashes, sinus problems, wheezing, and fatigue.

On the opposite end of the spectrum is *Stachybotrys Chartarum* (AKA Black Mold/Toxic Mold). This bad boy is more inclined to cause symptoms of brain fog, anxiety, stubborn weight gain, irritability, depression, and even anger. This is by no means a complete list. Again, much of it is reliant on the individual's immune system.

For many, the battle with mold is relentless and exhausting. To add to the problem, people are now spending more of their time cooped up inside their homes. According to the Environmental Protection Agency, the average person now spends **92%** of their time indoors!

Throw into the mix a house crammed with vinyl flooring, carpets, curtains, and paint. In a confined space, furniture stuffed with polyurethane foam irritates humans. They do so by off-gassing Volatile Organic Compounds (VOCs). Not surprisingly, 25 million Americans are currently dealing with asthma.

All too often, new building codes are slanted towards energy conservation. This has resulted in the tightening of building envelopes. With windows seldom in use, the amount of fresh air being exchanged is significantly reduced.

At this point, adding toxic mold to the list can send even the most robust immune system into a tailspin. Without wanting to sound like a broken record, anytime your home makes you feel sick, you should leave. Trying to heal in the same environment that made you ill will always be a challenge.

With that in mind, the rest of this book is geared towards practical mold solutions for the home, rather than personal detox protocols. Until your home is relatively free of mold, there is little point in trying to detoxify it.

Chapter 3: Ten molds you don't want to find in your home

To help us tackle molds, we must first know what they are. Molds are fungi, the plural of fungus. So far, their numbers have exceeded man's ability to count them. But one thing is for sure, wherever we go, there's a fungus among us.

Fortunately, we don't have to count their numbers. We only have to know which ones have the potential to cause us harm. As a rule of thumb, treat any unidentified mold with caution, but be especially wary of green molds. Ironically, *Stachybotrys*, often referred to as "black mold," isn't black at all, it's more of a dark greenish-black. It's also got a sticky film but I wouldn't recommend touching it.

Colors and sticky stuff aside, we can also split molds into three main categories. These are allergenic, pathogenic, and toxigenic. Some species can also cross over into one or more categories.

Allergenic

Allergenic molds cause the immune system to overreact. For people with a known allergy, itchy eyes, sneezing, and coughing are all too common. Mold allergies have also been linked to asthma. Asthma will cause wheezing, shortness of breath, and chest tightness. Some of the common molds in this category are *Alternaria, Aspergillus, Cladosporium*, and *Penicillium*.

Pathogenic

Pathogenic molds are opportunistic. Generally speaking, a person in good health can fight off most pathogenic molds. Those caught in the crosshairs are folks with suppressed or weakened immune systems. As we mentioned earlier, this makes infants and the elderly particularly susceptible. Pathogenic molds are also a cause for concern to anyone suffering from an acute illness. Pathogenic molds are commonly found in water-damaged homes.

Toxigenic

Unlike allergenic and pathogenic molds, toxigenic type molds do cause harm to humans. Toxigenic molds produce those poisonous chemicals known as mycotoxins. Prolonged exposure to mycotoxins, either at home or in the workplace, can lead to serious health problems.

Regardless of which type of mold you come up against, it's advisable to have it tested. This can be done with the help of a mold professional or, you can buy a DIY test kit. Both of these options are covered in the next chapter.

It's a common misconception that mold will only thrive in cold, damp climates. To be clear, mold can flourish in Arizona as easily as it can in Vermont. No matter which state you live in, if your home has a source of moisture (such as indoor plumbing) mold can exploit it.

With that in mind, here are ten molds you can find in any home. Each of them has the potential to cause health problems. The good news is, once you know what you are up against, your chances of dealing with it dramatically improve. Let's kick-off with *Stachybotrys*, AKA black mold/toxic mold.

1: STACHYBOTRYS

Stachybotrys thrives on damp, porous surfaces. Basements, laundry rooms, and bathrooms are all areas *Stachybotrys* will look to get a foothold. So long as there's excess moisture, *Stachybotrys* isn't too fussy about what it eats. Damp carpets, drywall, paper, cardboard, wicker baskets, you name it, *Stachybotrys* will find a way to destroy it.

Stachybotrys reproduces by releasing spores into the air. Like most mold spores, they can lay dormant for long periods. Given the right conditions, *Stachybotrys* also can produce mycotoxins. It all depends on the temperature, humidity, and surface that *Stachybotrys* is growing on.

Stachybotrys has a potent smell to it, sometimes described as musty, damp, or stale. The stronger the smell, the more developed the mold has become. In some cases, it can smell a lot like rotting wood. For this reason, *Stachybotrys* is usually uncovered by its smell long before it is seen.

Stachybotrys doesn't mind bad company. It will nearly always occur alongside other molds such as *Aspergillus* or *Cladosporium*.

Stachybotrys is—Allergenic/pathogenic/toxigenic.

2: ASPERGILLUS

There are roughly one hundred, and eighty different species of *Aspergillus*. They come in all shapes, sizes, and colors. Not surprisingly, they can be found in many American households. Although *Aspergillus* is listed as an allergenic mold, it certainly has the potential to turn toxic. This depends on the species. Some *Aspergillus* molds are also thought to produce aflatoxins.

Different *Aspergillus* types affect people in different ways. Allergy type symptoms are common. Although respiratory inflammation and asthma attacks have also been reported. In some cases, the lungs become infected leading to a disease known as *Aspergillosis*.

Aspergillosis is—Allergenic/pathogenic/toxigenic (depending on the species).

3: PENICILLIN

Penicillin has been used in medicine since 1942. As an antibiotic, this mold is generally considered safe. But as with any allergenic, Penicillin has the potential to cause a reaction.

Penicillin growing in the home can heap misery on a person. All the usual symptoms of coughing, sneezing, itchy eyes, etc. are present. If exposure is prolonged, it can also lead to chronic sinusitis. For people with immune disorders, symptoms may develop into further health complications. Pulmonary inflammation and asthma are common.

Often associated with water-damaged buildings, Penicillin is quick to spread. Hence, it's important to tackle any leaks as soon as possible. Left to its own devices, Penicillin will feed on carpets, curtains, cardboard, and even bedding. Wherever there is food and excess moisture, Penicillin will thrive!

Penicillin is—Allergenic.

4: FUSARIUM

Water-damaged homes seem to be a magnet for molds and *Fusarium* is no exception. For good measure, this one is capable of growing in cold temperatures. It's also allergenic *and* toxigenic.

Once *Fusarium* is detected, be sure to check all sections of the property. This one is a fast spreader and likes to move from room to room.

Exposure can lead to all the standard allergic-type reactions. Sore throat, running nose, sneezing, and itchy eyes. *Fusarium* is also capable of causing skin infections leading to dermatitis. It can even produce toxins that are damaging to the nervous system. In susceptible individuals, prolonged exposure may cause severe and life-threatening conditions.

Like all molds, *Fusarium* will feed on porous materials. Drywall, wallpaper, wood, carpet, curtains, or other fabrics, etc. Reducing clutter can help reduce the spread.

Fusarium is—Allergenic/pathogenic/toxigenic.

5: CLADOSPORIUM

Cladosporium is adaptable, it can thrive in both hot and cold and climates. It also likes to hide under floorboards and inside wardrobes. It has a suede-like texture with an olive-green or brown colored mold. It can grow on indoor fabrics such as carpets, curtains, upholstery, etc.

As an allergenic, you can expect to experience watery eyes, an itchy throat, runny nose, and in some cases, skin irritation. Prolonged exposure may lead to sinusitis, asthma, and lung infections. *Cladosporium*, like all suspect molds, should not be handled without protective equipment.

Cladosporium is—Allergenic/pathogenic.

6: ACREMONIUM

Acremonium is a group of approximately one hundred and fifty different molds. Some are harmless while others are toxigenic and pathogenic.

With a slightly higher demand for moisture, *Acremonium* is well suited to leaky buildings. They also thrive in water-damaged homes, schools, offices, and public buildings.

Due to its thirsty nature, *Acremonium* is sometimes found in air conditioning units. Other places to keep an eye on are windowsills, laundry rooms, bathrooms, basements, and below sinks where leaks often develop.

Over time, *Acremonium* may change in appearance. It starts out as a small, moist mold but turns into a fine powdery substance. *Acremonium* molds can be grey, pink, orange, or white in color. Like most molds, it has an affinity for porous materials. It will grow just fine on drywall, wallpaper, and plywood, etc.

Some of the pathogenic species of *Acremonium* have the power to cause infections. These infections can be classified as superficial, locally invasive, or disseminated. The latter refers to an infection that has spread throughout an entire organ or body.

Acremonium can also cause onychomycosis (an infection of the nails). Other species are known to colonize the lungs. This can result in a growth known as a pulmonary fungal ball. Just to keep you on your toes, many of these symptoms can overlap. As always, so much of this is dependent on the strength of a person's immune system. Symptoms may also present themselves as allergies, hay fever, or asthma.

Acremonium is—Allergenic/pathogenic/toxigenic.

7: MUCOR

Mucor is another thirsty mold. It likes to hang out in air conditioner units, HVAC systems, and bathrooms. Pretty much any place where moisture is elevated. *Mucor* is usually white or greyish in color and grows in thick patches.

Be careful with this one, it's another fast spreader and has an affinity for the respiratory system. Difficulty breathing, fever, and flu-like symptoms are all common. *Mucor* can also make existing asthma conditions worse.

In severe cases, *mucormycosis* can develop. *Mucormycosis* (previously called *zygomycosis*) is a serious fungal infection. It can damage the lungs, sinuses, and even the brain. It can also infect the nose and eyes eventually becoming systemic in the blood. This can have an impact on other internal systems. For this reason, it's important not to handle *Mucor* spores without the correct safety equipment. We'll cover protective equipment later in the book.

    Mucor—Allergenic/pathogenic

8: TRICHODERMA

Trichoderma is an allergenic mold type with five different subspecies. Primarily, it's a soil-dwelling fungi but it's highly adaptable. Like all molds, it thrives in moist areas. It can be found chilling out on damp carpets, curtains, wallpaper, or other fabrics. You might also find it in air conditioning filters or the ductwork of your HVAC system.

Trichoderma is generally white in color with green patches. These are fast-growing molds and can be found as wooly-textured clusters. Over time, these clusters become more compact.

Although listed as an allergenic, some *Trichoderma* molds can produce mycotoxins. It can act a lot like *Stachybotrys*.

Trichoderma contains an enzyme that destroys wood and paper products. Given its ability to spread, *Trichoderma* can weaken the structure of a building.

Trichoderma is—Allergenic/pathogenic/toxigenic

9: ULOCLADIUM

Ulocladium is no stranger to water-damaged buildings. It can also be found wherever condensation is rampant such as bathrooms.

Ulocladium also likes moldy company. It has no problem teaming up with *Stachybotrys*, *Chromium*, and *Fusarium*. As a rule of thumb, the presence of Ulocladium is a good indicator of water damage. It has a suede-like texture and can be brown, gray, or greenish-black in color.

Ulocladium has two different subspecies of molds. Both can cause health problems. General asthma type symptoms and difficulty breathing being the most common. Some report skin infections and hay fever-type reactions.

Ulocladium is—Allergenic/pathogenic

10: CHAETOMIUM

Chaetomium has a cotton-texture to it. As it matures, it goes from white to gray to brown. It then turns black. What sets *Chaetomium* apart from other molds is its unique, musty odor.

Chaetomium enjoys damp, warm conditions. It can be found in poorly ventilated attics especially homes with leaky roofs. But it can also thrive in damp basements, or areas prone to water spillages such as sinks and shower areas.

Chaetomium is both allergenic and toxigenic. Like most allergenic molds, it has the potential to cause respiratory issues, skin lesions, and infections of the sinuses and lungs. Be sure not to touch this one without gloves as it can lead to skin and nail infections.

Chaetomium is—Allergenic/pathogenic/toxigenic.

HIT THE WEAK POINT

Reading through this list you may have come to the conclusion that mold is a formidable opponent. It is, but that doesn't mean it's infallible. All living things have a weakness. In case you missed it, mold needs three things to stay alive, food, water, and humidity.

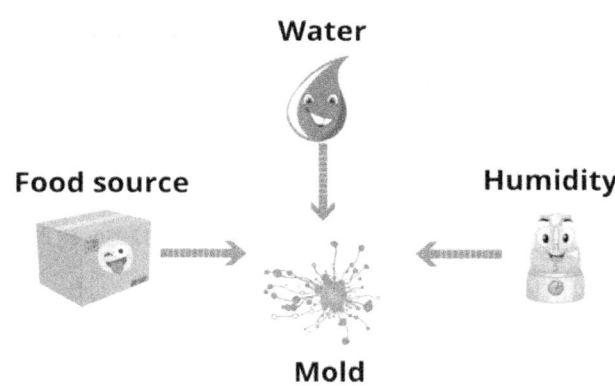

Dealing with an outbreak of mold can be overwhelming at the best of times, I get it. But if we break the problem down into three manageable parts, it becomes easier to process. You can strike at the heart of mold by controlling any one of these three things, food, water, or humidity. So, don't give up. Now that you understand the problem, successful mold remediation becomes easier to achieve.

Chapter 4: How to test your home for mold

Finding a mold test is pretty easy. But as always, the devil is in the details. Some tests can be a waste of money; others can give a false sense of security. So before spending a dime of your hard-earned cash, let's begin with a few tests that cost no money at all but can work like a charm. We'll then dive a little deeper and see which mold tests offer the best value for money.

FREE TEST

We can use our nose to sniff out mold (intended pun). Some molds have a stale, musty odor to them. Over time, homeowners may even get used to the smell. Or even worse, they try to cover it over with air-freshener!

As a rule, if a room smells funky then suspect mold. Remember, *Stachybotrys* (AKA black mold) has a potent musty smell to it as does *Chaetomium*.

We can also rely on our immune system to detect mold. As we learned earlier, symptoms of coughing, sneezing, wheezing are commonplace. If your doctor hasn't been able to pinpoint the cause of your "mystery" allergy, it might be time to have your home tested for mold.

Moving along nicely, we can use our eyes to check walls and ceilings for signs of mold. It likes to hide behind watermarks and comes in different shapes and colors.

With that housework out of the way, let us now enter the weird and wonderful world of testing. We'll start with the least expensive option first.

$10 TESTS

Most hardware stores sell a DIY test kit for as little as $10. It consists of a petri dish and a growing solution. While this type of test may be a good starting point, it's not intended to cover all molds. Think of it as a mousetrap for mold.

The solution is added to the petri dish and then placed in a suspect area for twenty-four hours. Once the time is up, close the lid, and watch for signs of mold growth. At this point, don't be too alarmed when you see mold sprouting. As we have already discovered, just about every home/workplace has mold spores present.

Now that you have a fresh crop of mold, the next question is, what are you going to do with it?

Well, if you wanted to impress people, it serves as a great visual aid to show people your home has a mold issue. I'm thinking of doubting landlords as opposed to random strangers. Generally speaking, the latter would just be weird.

Most homeowners send the sample off to a lab for testing. Don't worry, the address details come with the kit. For this service, you can expect to pay an extra fee along with the shipping. Typically, this will bump the price up to around $60.

Although this approach is cheap and cheerful, some users complain that kits have no sell-by date. In theory, the sterile petri dish may have been sitting on the hardware shelves for any amount of time. In some cases, this could lead to your lab results being skewed.

OTHER TESTS

Other forms of self-tests are tape lift test, swab test, and bulk test. The tape test is the hardest one to mess up. Simply peel back the tape, stick onto a suspect mold, mark the sample, and send it to the lab. Again, you can expect to pay extra for the lab results.

Swabs test, as the name suggests, are swabbed over a suspect area. The sample is then sealed, labeled, and sent to the lab for analysis. For this test, you can again expect to pay upwards of $60.

Bulk samples are a little different. They are usually cut from a suspect area. This could be a piece of wood, drywall, or any other building material contaminated with mold. This method requires careful attention as disturbing mold can prompt it to spread. Once the sample has been collected, it is then placed in a plastic Ziploc bag and sent to a lab.

If you are just starting out, these types of tests are relatively inexpensive and do have merit to them. But it's not possible to accurately gauge mold levels with a single test kit. It's best to think of these tests as single pieces to a larger puzzle.

Superior results come by combining the above tests with an air sample. An air sample sucks air into the mouth of an open cartridge. For this option, you may need an extra piece of equipment. Some DIY kits have been adapted to use a regular vacuum cleaner.

To establish a baseline, an outdoor air sample is taken and then compared to an indoor sample. Additional samples are then taken from one or more suspect rooms. Depending on how many rooms you have, this can become expensive quicker than a speeding ticket. The true cost may even exceed bringing in a professional.

ERMI

The ERMI (Environmental Relative Moldiness Index) test is popular with many in the natural health field. Most swear by it claiming that it detects molds other tests may have missed. It costs around $300 and uses dust samples taken from carpets. The kit comes with an attachment that fits directly to the hose of a standard vacuum cleaner. Once you have your sample, ERMI will then use a DNA-based method to identify thirty-six different species of mold. So far so good, but what if you don't have a carpet?

In uncarpeted areas, a Swiffer cloth can be used to collect dust samples. Although from the lab's perspective, this is treated as a separate test and you can expect to pay an extra fee. When it comes to mold testing, ain't nothing for nothing.

HERTSMI-2

This test works similarly to the one above, dust samples are collected and analyzed for mold. The main difference is the price. A HERTSMI-2 test will set you back around $125 but the tradeoff is that you only get tested for five mold species.

With more than 100,000 species of mold to choose from, it's unrealistic for any test to pick up on every species. What we don't want to find is dangerous molds at high levels.

CHAIN OF CUSTODY

While researching this book, I took the time to read some of the Amazon reviews for the DIY kits. In some cases, there seemed to be an element of inconsistency with the lab results. Areas with no mold have come back positive, and just as worrying, areas with a known mold issue have come back clear. I can only speculate that the reason for this is a breakdown in the chain of custody (also known as COC). This has to do with the way samples are collected and labeled.

To make this point, have you ever been to a restaurant where the server got your order wrong? Perhaps he/she wrote it down wrong, or perhaps the duty chef read it wrong. Either way, your fried lobster now looks a lot like a tuna sandwich. Obviously, somebody, somewhere in the chain got confused.

In the mold industry, a COC form records the movement of samples. This begins at the point of collection and ends in the hands of an eager lab technician.

When the COC form is filled out correctly, you can expect to see accurate results. But a simple slip of the pen and your results will be about as much use as a wooden frying pan.

Are there other tests on the market? Yes, lots, but the aim of this chapter isn't to overwhelm you, it's to inform you of the options. Whenever somebody is selling a test, it's important to look at things objectionably. Personally, I'm not selling you anything which helps to keep me unbiased.

So, which do I think is best?

Well, that kinda depends. If you are on a tight budget, I can appreciate that your options are limited. If this is the case, then the least expensive test is better than no test at all. That said, there is no point in spending good money on tests unless the root cause of your mold issue has been found and fixed. Don't panic, there's a checklist later in the book to help you do this.

However, if you are thinking about spending three or four hundred bucks on testing, then my advice is to use a licensed mold inspector. Ideally, find one who has zero interest in doing remedial work. This prevents any conflict of interest.

At the time of writing, professional mold inspections start at around $400. This isn't a million miles away from some of the DIY tests. Especially when you factor in all those sneaky, hidden costs. Although you can expect to pay more for larger properties.

Another advantage with mold inspectors is they conduct multiple testing. This usually begins with an air test and is then backed up with swab samples or a tape lift. Additionally, they can also call upon specialized thermal imaging equipment. This allows the inspector to check for leaks behind walls.

Over time, an experienced mold inspector will develop an intuition for mold. This can help lead them to areas of your home you may not have thought of. Hiring a mold inspector also ensures that the COC is filled out correctly.

When hiring *any* professional, use someone local, and don't be afraid to ask for references.

Chapter 5: PPE for mold

As Mother Nature's great recycler, mold has been with us since the beginning of time. It continues to thrive thanks to its superpower, namely, a blast of mycotoxins to the face.

Attempting to treat mold without a plan is like jumping out of an airplane without a parachute. Ideally, large infestations are best handled by professionals. But an informed homeowner should be able to tackle smaller outbreaks with success. The key is to act quickly, the longer mold is left to fester, the more damage it causes.

As a rule of thumb, if the moldy area is easy to access, and less than ten square feet (that's roughly 3 ft. x 3 ft.), then it's a doable project. But there are a few safety precautions to be taken into consideration.

PPE

We've heard a lot about PPE (Personal Protective Equipment) during the 2020 pandemic. Face masks, hazmat suits, and gloves all became a common sight.

You may have noticed how the lab technicians in Wuhan dressed like they were handling plutonium. While some folks here in the US felt that a bandana offered the same level of protection. My point is this, any threat, be it from a microscopic virus, or a teeny-weeny mold spore has to be matched with the right equipment. When it comes to toxic mold, covering your face with a paper face mask provides a false sense of security.

This chapter aims to provide a rundown of the different types of PPE that are available. This will help form an effective barrier between you and mold. As always, I have zero affiliation with any of the products I mention, I'm simply trying to save you some time.

To keep mold spores out of the eyes, nose, and mouth, a full-face respirator offers the most protection. If you know you are susceptible to mold, I'm writing this for you.

Handling dangerous molds is a tricky business. With that in mind, it's best to air on the side of caution. A full-face respirator will set you back approximately $150. If price is an issue, feel free to shop around. There are lots of other masks on the market. That said, the Moldex 9000 full-face respirator is a pretty good one. It's also less expensive than a trip to the doctor ... *just saying*.

On either side of the face mask, is a canister which acts as filters. Canisters are removable and can be changed to meet different hazards. When dealing with mold, pay attention to the numbers written on the front of the canister. P100 HEPA filters ensure that 99.7% of particles larger than 0.3 microns are filtered out.

THE HALF MASK

As the name suggests, a half mask only covers half of the face. It's also half the price which makes an attractive option. Any money you might save is worth spending on a set of goggles. Note: Goggles are not safety glasses. Safety glasses have large gaps around the edges which give spores access to the eyes.

The Nasum M201 is a pretty good half-face respirator. It's also certified for professional use. The filters on either side of the M201 include a carbon layer that reduces the number of particles you breathe in.

At the time of writing, a mold rated half-mask costs around $40. A slightly less expensive option can be found in some hardware stores.

Again, the numbers written on the filter tell a story. P100 filters will filter out 99.7% of particles. Once opened, P100 filters should last around six months. The good news is, once you have the mask, replacing the filters is inexpensive and easy to do.

Half-masks come in medium, and large so be sure to get your size. A mask can only offer protection if it fits properly. When you finish using it, take the mask outside and wipe it clean. Always store it in a dry place away from any mold source.

N-95 MASKS

Your least expensive option is an N-95 particulate respirator (AKA, the paper mask). These can be a little stuffy to wear and are not recommended for anyone with breathing issues. Issues such as Chronic Obstructive Pulmonary Disease (COPD) or asthma. Some N-95 models have a valve on the front that makes breathing easier

To work as intended, N-95 respirators must fit properly. Those with facial hair are unlikely to get any benefit from wearing one. N95 respirators offer zero protection against chemicals or gases such as Carbon Monoxide.

The N-95 *isn't* meant for long term use and should never be shared. Think of it as disposable protection. Fortunately, a box of ten sells for approx. $12 (good luck finding one of those in the middle of a pandemic).

The "N-95" number stamped on the front relates to its ability to block out particles. An N–95 mask is intended to stop ninety-five percent of particles 0.3 microns in size or larger. As with the half-mask, eyes must be protected with goggles.

GLOVES AND CLOTHES

When dealing with mold, long, rubber gloves that cover the forearms are recommended. This will help protect the skin from the mold as well as any chemicals that might irritate the skin.

If you are susceptible to mold, it's worth spending $10 on a disposable hazmat suit. These will cover the head, ears, and clothes. Once the project is complete, simply dispose of the hazmat suit in a plastic bag. This will help to stop mold spores from contaminating other areas of the property.

If you decide to skip the hazmat suit, be sure to wash your clothes as soon as the job is complete. As we mentioned earlier, adding an EC3 to the washing machine can help kill off any mold spores.

For smaller, less toxic projects, you could try adding Borax to the wash instead. Borax is a naturally occurring mineral that's been mined for hundreds of years. It's safe to mix with laundry detergents and is sometimes used to boost their cleaning power.

Wearing old clothes that you don't mind throwing away is another option.

With all our PPE ducks nicely in a row, we can now move forward with the task in hand—our first mold remediation project!

Ready?

Chapter 6: Why bleach rarely works but this will

One of the earliest mold remediation protocols dates back to the Old Testament. It goes something like this ...

If the mold has spread in the house, it is a persistent defiling mold; the house is unclean. It must be torn down, its stones, timbers, and all the plaster—taken out of the town to an unclean place.—Leviticus 14

Today, we take a different approach to mold removal but the fundamentals remain the same. This chapter will guide you through the process and help you stop mold in its tracks.

Some mold outbreaks are easier to fix than others. If mold is growing on a removable item (like a carpet) simply adopt the biblical principle and throw it out. This will save you hours of wasted time and unmatched levels of stress. Why not do it now, while it's fresh in your mind?

Mold growing on a hard surface is pretty easy to deal with too. Hard surfaces prevent mold from getting a grip with its invasive root system. This makes plastic items, sinks, bathtubs, window frames, and ceramic items, ideal candidates. You can scrub the mold off a hard surface using one of the following solutions.

THE UNNATURAL APPROACH

On hard surfaces, bleach is inexpensive and easy to use. But it can also irritate skin, lungs, and eyes. Any time you use bleach, remember to ventilate the room. Never mix bleach with ammonia. When the two are combined, they release gases that cause damage to the lungs. With that in mind, it's probably best to use something less toxic.

THE NATURAL APPROACH (it's not what you think)

For hard surfaces, distilled, white vinegar kills 82% of molds. Compared to bleach, it's also much safer and just as inexpensive. To get rid of mold, pour undiluted vinegar into a spray bottle. Spray the area, leave for an hour, and wipe clean. Hey presto, mold be gone!

Baking soda works pretty well also. It can be mixed with white vinegar to make a powerful, mold-busting paste. Mix two parts baking soda, with one-part vinegar, and one-part water. Once it becomes a thick paste, spread it over the mold and allow it to dry. Once the paste is scrubbed off, it takes the mold with it. Best of all, nobody has to get sick from toxic chemicals.

Top marks, for slaying mold like a pro. But let's not get too ahead of ourselves, we still have to tackle those porous mold problems. *Here's where it gets tricky ...*

Side note: When mold is growing on porous materials, neither bleach nor vinegar will have little impact on it.

POROUS MATERIALS

Anything that used to be a tree is a porous material. Items such as cardboard boxes, newspapers, and wicker baskets, etc. are pretty easy to pick up and throw out. But what happens if the porous material is the 2x6 timber holding up a part of your ceiling, roof, or sub-floor?

Well, the first thing we need to ask is where is the mold getting its moisture from? If it's a leaking roof, window, or pipe, then you need to find it and fix it. No matter how well you treat the mold, it'll always come back and bite you on the bum if you don't have control of the source of water/moisture.

For now, let's imagine your eagle-like eye has just spotted a brown watermark on your bedroom ceiling. Oddly enough, there's also a musty smell in the room that has been making you sneeze and wheeze. In my book, that sounds a lot like mold. So before reaching for the stain blocking paint, it might be a good idea to fix that leak.

Aha! Leak found, a plumber is called, and the leak is fixed, problem over, right? Meh, not so fast, Tonto. While the plumber has a hole cut in your ceiling it's worth grabbing a flashlight and checking for signs of wetness. (On the 2x6 timbers, not the plumber).

If on closer inspection you find the 2x6 is wet or damp (but free of mold), then let the area dry out before sealing it back up. All too often, plumbers skip this step (plumbers are good like that) and the moisture has nowhere to go. This creates a fertile breeding ground for microscopic mold spores to feed on.

Okay, let's back up and imagine a different scenario. This time, your leak has been fixed but on closer inspection, you notice a mold-like substance is growing on the drywall.

REMEMBER THE 3 x 3 RULE

If the mold problem looks bigger than 3ft x 3ft, it's best to stop what you are doing and call for backup. Just as you called a plumber to fix the leak, a mold inspector can help you assess the mold problem. Lest we forget, larger mold outbreaks have a nasty habit of spreading.

However, if your moldy ceiling project is under 3ft x 3ft and you'd like to tackle the project yourself, here's how you do it ...

First, you have to decide what level of PPE you will need. If your health is in pretty good shape, you might be able to get away with wearing a mask and goggles. But if you are on your last legs, it's best to go all-in with a full-face respirator, gloves, goggles, and a hazmat suit. Once you have the correct PPE, you can then tackle the project in hand.

Okay, given that our imaginary drywall has mold sprouting out of it, it needs to be cut out and sent to the dump. To do this safely, there are a few simple steps involved in the process.

SHUT IT OFF

Mold doesn't take kindly to being cut out of its home (AKA, your ceiling). In a last-ditch attempt to save itself, the mold is gonna attempt to dump some of its mold spores. With that in mind, it's a good idea to shut off the HVAC system (Heating, Ventilation, and Air Conditioning). The last thing we need is all those tiny spores getting sucked into the works. Once they become airborne, it's hard to know which direction they could get blown in.

NOW, SEAL IT OFF

Before disturbing the mold, it's best to seal off the room you are working in. This can be done with inexpensive plastic sheeting from the hardware store.

If you have a couple of jacks to hold up the plastic sheeting, more power to you. If not, you don't need anything fancy, painters' tape will hold it up to the ceiling and walls. Take your time with this step, you don't want the plastic sheeting to fall halfway through the job. That would suck.

If there's a window in the room, open it. At this point, an inexpensive fan comes in handy. Have it blowing outward on a low setting. This will create negative air pressure inside the room. Negative air pressure simply means you are sucking the air out of the room. With the help of the plastic sheeting, any stray mold spores will go out of the window. Hoorah for negative air pressure!

With the area now sealed off, and your fan in place, it's time to cut out that moldy drywall. Remember, mold has an extensive root system that can penetrate far and wide. We don't want to miss any of the mold so it's best to cut out a little extra on either side. Trust me, nobody wants to do this kind of project twice because they missed a spot.

The easiest way to do this is to mark the area with a pencil. But allow an extra 2ft all around for good measure. Use the pencil mark to guide you. Then, score the pencil line with a sharp utility knife.

At all times, work slowly and carefully. If the drywall is pretty damp, you may find it crumbles into pieces. Either way, place the moldy drywall into plastic bags and seal them up. This will cut down on any cross-contamination as you drag them through the house.

Once you have the moldy drywall bagged up, remove any insulation in the area and bag that up, too (the paper on the back of the insulation is something mold likes to snack on). Having enough plastic bags on hand saves walking through the home looking for more. As my old drill sergeant used to say, "Proper Planning Prevents Poor Performance." He called it his five P rule, lol.

With the drywall and insulation out of the way, it's time to inspect the surrounding timbers. If it's dry, add new insulation, apply fresh drywall, and wait for family members to shower you with praise. Seriously, you deserve a pat on the back for a job well done.

However, it's not uncommon to find the mold has spread to the surrounding timbers. At this point, those same family members may now take a step back from you and question your mental state for taking on such a project. Don't panic, oh bold one, every problem has a solution.

If the timber *is* damp and rotting, then simply cut it out. No need to make a big song and dance about it. You can either hire a carpenter to do it or, if you are pretty handy, cut it back yourself. As with the drywall, just take off a little extra for good measure. If it helps, there are lots of DIY carpentry videos on YouTube.

To be fair, that's the worst-case scenario. Most of the time the timbers are solid and perhaps just a little damp or show signs of surface mold. Both of these problems are treatable, but please, not with bleach. If anything, bleach will make matters worse. A much better option is to use an antimicrobial. An antimicrobial is a liquid agent that can either kill microorganisms or stop their growth.

There are lots of antimicrobial products on the market. Concrobium Mold Control is a pretty good one. It's also easy to find as most hardware stores carry it. Concrobium is odorless and contains no harmful chemicals or Volatile Organic Compounds (VOCs). This makes it a good choice for those who are sensitive to harsh chemicals.

For small projects, Concrobium comes in its own spray bottle. For larger areas, add Concrobium to a garden pump sprayer. You can usually pick one of these up for under $10 at a hardware store. Concrobium sells for around $30 a gallon. There's no need to dilute it, pour it straight into the container and spray. Once the area has been treated, let it soak in overnight.

DRY OUT

Before you seal everything back up, check that the area has dried out. A dehumidifier can help speed the drying process up. If you don't own a dehumidifier, you can rent them out by the day.

If in doubt, you can always double-check how dry the timber is with a moisture meter. This is a handy little gadget that retails online for about $25. Just pop the two prongs onto *any* surface and it'll give you an instant moisture reading.

Before you wrap it up, it wouldn't hurt to run over the area with a HEPA rated vacuum cleaner. This is important as some mycotoxins that fall to the floor are allergenic and will continue to be a source of toxicity.

So long as the HEPA filter is fitted correctly, and the seals aren't worn, it will capture 99.97% of dead mold spores and mycotoxins.

Remember, a successful mold removal project is a one-two approach. It's not enough to just kill the mold, dead spores and mycotoxins are best removed. HEPA filters have been doing this kind of thing for eighty plus years.

Now that we know how to contain and remove mold from drywall, what say we take on a different project? This next one causes more problems than any other place in the home. It is, of course, the very foundation your home sits on!

Chapter 7: The hidden danger inside your basement — Wooden pallets!

Over the years, I seem to have spent a lot of my spare time in other people's basements. Whenever I see wooden pallets, it tells me that the homeowner has a problem with mold. *How so?*

People place wooden pallets on basement floors to keep cardboard boxes dry. Here's the thing, if the basement floor has enough moisture to make cardboard boxes damp, then it has enough moisture for mold to grow on the wooden pallet. This *will* quickly spread to the contents of the cardboard box. Contents such as soft toys, clothes, documents, holiday decorations, bedding, etc. I can't tell you why people feel the need to store pillows in a damp basement, but I can assure you they do. Pillows, like all forms of bedding, are porous which makes them an ideal food for mold to munch on. If a picture is worth a thousand words, *this* is what I'm talking about.

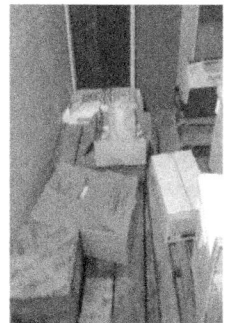 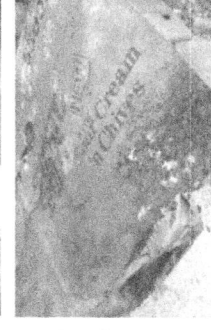 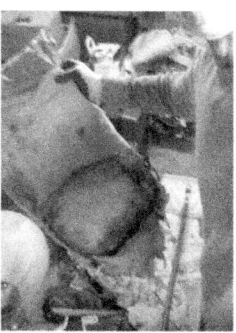

BOXES ON PALLETS   MOLD ON THE BOX   PILLOW IN THE BOX

At some point, cardboard boxes (along with any mold spores) have a way of finding their way back into the main house. Who knows, perhaps even in a kid's bedroom. Now we have two problems, shall we go for three?

When the child gets sick from mold, doctors will rarely make the connection to a moldy basement. It's simply not on their radar. With that in mind, one of the most effective ways to prevent the spread of mold is to keep your basement free of clutter. No carpets, no furniture, no cuddly toys, no bedding, nothing, zilch, nada.

Basements are a magnet for junk. You know it, and I know it. If it wasn't junk, it wouldn't be sitting in a dark, moldy basement on a pallet. In case you are still wondering what I have against wooden pallets, this is how they look when they are flipped over.

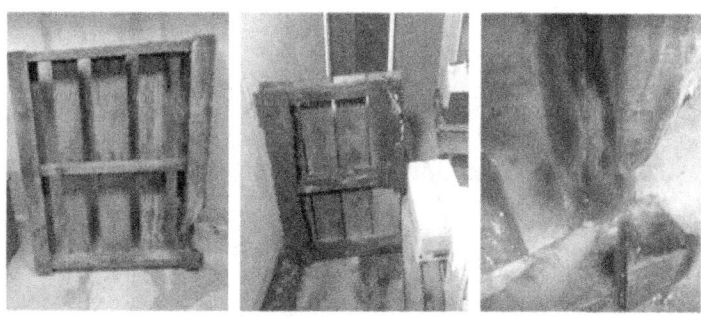

Trust me on this one, adopting a minimalist approach will serve you better than owning a basement full of "stuff".

Once you come to terms with letting go of your clutter, dispose of it carefully. Offloading it onto someone else only gives them the problem. This is something to keep in mind whenever you see that "bargain" at a yard sale. The chances are, you are bringing home a new strain of mold. I hate to break it to you, but the best place to send basement clutter is to the landfill.

Seeing a dumpster parked on your driveway is a great source of motivation. It's almost uncanny how it helps you to say goodbye to all that old junk. The stuff you thought you needed but deep down you know you never will.

Once you have your basement back under your control, you'll want to dry it out. All that stale, damp air is best directed outside and a set of high-powered fans may help the cause. Obviously, any fan needs to be aimed directly out of an open window rather than blowing mold spores around. Depending on how much moisture you are trying to move, a commercial-grade dehumidifier is a better tool for this. Alas, buying a decent one comes at considerable expense. But you can check with your local hardware store, they usually have them for hire.

However, if your basement has a dirt floor then a dehumidifier is going to be as much use to you as a chocolate teapot. There's just too much moisture coming up from the ground. The only way to fix this problem is to have the area sealed with a layer of concrete. Before concrete is poured, the area should be sealed with a layer of Visqueen (thick black plastic). This stops any damp from coming up under the concrete.

If funds are a little tight, start with the layer of thick plastic. This can be an inexpensive, short term fix. When laying down the thick, black plastic, make sure that it doesn't have any gaps. This will defeat the objective causing damp to escape and travel upwards.

Whenever possible, it's best to get the plastic sheet down in one piece. Failing that, overlap any joins and weigh them down with bricks. Trying to glue seams on a damp floor isn't going to happen. Once the basement floor is sealed, (either with concrete or a layer of thick plastic) you can then extract moisture from the air with a dehumidifier.

If mold has already taken hold in your basement, you may need to treat the area with an antimicrobial agent. If the mold has spread to an area that's bigger than 3ft x 3ft, you should make a call to your local mold inspector. A mold inspector can help you access the severity of the problem. All things being equal, let's take a look at what else you may have going on in your basement.

HVAC

HVAC systems (Heating, Ventilation, and Air Conditioning) are designed to balance indoor air temperatures. As a rule, you'll need to hire a professional to service this equipment. But that doesn't mean you can't poke your head inside to look for signs of mold. Depending on what you discover, it may be necessary to have your HVAC system professionally cleaned and sanitized.

If your home is heated with forced hot air via a furnace, check that the ductwork is sealed properly. Any gaps or cracks will allow stale basement air/mold to be sucked up and blow around your living room. If you live in an apartment building, HVAC systems have the potential to spread mold throughout an entire building. I'm not telling you this to freak you out, I'm telling you because it might be something you overlook.

WASHER/DRYER

Doing your laundry in a basement is one way to get a daily hit of musty old mold. If you have space in your home, consider bringing the washer/drier up out of the basement. From a plumbing perspective, this is super easy to do.

Across Europe, most people do their laundry in a small room off the kitchen (AKA "the laundry room"). Compared to walking up and down basement steps (with a heavy washing basket), a laundry room is a safer, more efficient option.

Either way, hot air from the dryer needs to leave the home. A partially blocked vent pipe isn't just a fire hazard, it's a sure way to cause a rapid buildup of moisture.

CRAWLSPACES

To reduce construction costs, some homes (or sections of them) may have a crawl space under them. As the name suggests, a crawlspace has just enough room to crawl around in. Oftentimes, dirt and rocks are left in place, sometimes, just a few feet away from a living space. There's nothing wrong with this so long air can flow freely through the area.

With enough ventilation, the chances of mold working its way up to the living space are minimized. Hence, areas under decks are usually finished off with some kind of open latticework.

Problems develop whenever airflow is restricted in some way. In colder climates, this can happen when homeowners insulate their crawlspace. This is usually done to try and limit chilly wind factors. In case you missed it, mold spores like to grow in dirt. Once a crawlspace is enclosed it stifles airflow and mold can now work its way up into the living space.

Having the area "professionally" encapsulated has been known to work but it's not cheap. The other problem is finding good people to do the job right. Most old school builders are now retired. I'm not saying good people aren't still out there. But generally speaking, most folks coming into the construction industry don't want a career that involves crawling on their belly, and who could blame them?

If you are having crawl space issues, and need additional information, check out Crawlspaceninja.com. Michael Church, the owner, does good work and he's super knowledgeable. He's also put together a collection of free videos that you might find helpful.

If you are in the market for a new home, you could avoid many of these problems by finding a property *without* a basement/crawlspace. Until these types of moisture issues are resolved, mold will continue to plague the homeowner.

SUMP PUMPS

When it comes to keeping water out of a basement (or crawlspace), sump pumps play an interesting role. Here's the theory—water comes in, the pump kicks in, water gets pumped out, and life is good. But there's a problem, *can you see it?*

Sump pumps work on electricity. In the middle of a storm, it's not uncommon for a homeowner to lose power. With no pump, the basement then doubles up as an indoor swimming pool. However, this handy addition isn't what the homeowner's had in mind.

The solution to a failed pump is to install an expensive, battery backup system. This reminds me of a story I once heard about NASA scientists.

Legend has it, in the 1960's, NASA scientists realized that regular Earth pens wouldn't work in space. Millions of taxpayer dollars later, astronauts took to the sky with their new gravity-defying pens. Their Soviet counterparts took a slightly different approach. They simply handed them cosmonauts pencils. I don't know if that's true or not, but in my mind simple ideas *always* work better than complicated ones.

Perhaps it's a man thing, but when it comes to keeping water out of a basement, some contractors like to over complicate things. If only there was another way.

Wait a second, maybe there is!

Instead of pumping water out of the basement, what if we just stopped the water from coming in? It's a radical idea I know, but stay tuned, I'll show you how to do this in the following chapter for pennies on the dollar!

Chapter 8: How to Stop Basements Flooding

As the saying goes, "a boat is a hole in the water you throw money into." By the same token, it could be said that a basement is a hole under your house that fills up with water and problems.

At best, basements are a storage area for things we rarely need. At worst, they become a fertile breeding ground for toxic mold. Yet, there is a simple, inexpensive solution any homeowner can try. But first, why do we even need a basement?

Well, it might surprise you to know, many homes do fine without them. 99.9% of Australian homes don't have basements. Nor do the Japanese, who took it a step further, and in some places, basements are prohibited by law! Across Europe, many buildings have stood for hundreds of years without a basement.

Here in the US, the majority of homes on the West Coast are also basement free.

And yet, home builders on the East Coast and Midwest, continue to dig big holes and then plonk a third of the house into it. Some would argue that a house needs a basement to prevent the foundation from shifting.

Really?

Didn't we just cover how those crazy European foundations have withstood the test of time?

Yes, foundations need to be built below the frost line, this we can all agree on. But to say basements are essential to the integrity of the structure is simply not true. I grew up in a cold, damp part of England that was hit hard with snow every winter. To this day, that house is still standing and nope, it doesn't have a basement.

As you can probably tell, I'm not a huge fan of leaky basements. I've worked in construction for more than thirty years and I've yet to see a basement that doesn't leak. To add to the problem, basements can be a source of naturally occurring Radon. Radon is a tasteless, odorless gas that is difficult to detect. It also poses a serious health hazard. *I digress.*

For the past fifteen years, I've been living on the East Coast. This has given me ample opportunity to see plenty of leaky basements firsthand. I then put my British ingenuity to the test. The good news is, I found an inexpensive way to stop water from entering the basement.

It's no secret that basements have a nasty habit of flooding. Once the water gets in, it mixes with clutter which then becomes a magnet for mold. But where does all the water come from?

In a word, rainwater.

When rainwater gushes out of the sky, it lands on your roof. All things being equal, it will then enter the gutter system and head downwards. So far, so good.

But once the ground below becomes waterlogged, all that rainwater has nowhere to go but down. It doesn't take long for water to find the foundation.

Over time, foundations tend to develop hairline cracks. In the colder months, these tiny cracks fill up with water which then freezes.

This continues to play out until one day, those tiny cracks open up even more. Now, groundwater seeps into the basement usually, after a heavy rainstorm.

A pump is then installed. If it fails, homeowners will look to hire a contractor. Any contractor willing to go toe to toe with Mother Nature will turn up on site in a big red truck, wearing mirror sunglasses, and crocodile skin boots. It's just the way it is.

At considerable expense, a mechanical digger may also arrive on-site. Thousands of dollars later, a French drain is installed. And when that fails, homeowners get real pissed, real quick. Been there, seen it, got the T-shirt to prove it. Take a closer look at the problem ...

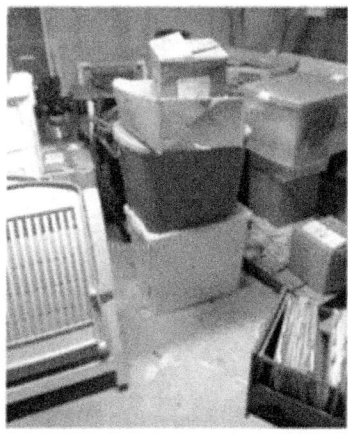 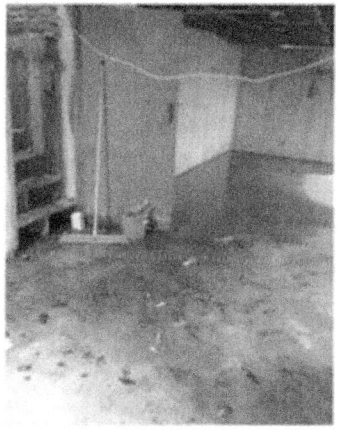

Perhaps you have also experienced the joys of moving clutter and carrying buckets of water out of your basement?

Rather than keep pumping water out, the said contractor may then decide to stop the water coming in. Yup, sounds like a plan to me.

At this point, the contractor will then have a truckload of fresh dirt delivered to your home. Next, he'll have his crew grade the dirt away from your house with a rake. At last, we seem to be on the right track but this new, bold approach has a flaw. *Can you see it?*

At first, that fresh layer of dirt *will* soak up rainwater like a giant sponge. But it doesn't take long before it too becomes waterlogged. Over time, this dirt may even wash away. So how do we stop the rainwater from doing this?

First, the entire area needs to be graded away from your home. Second, it has to be sealed, preferably with concrete. Concrete prevents rainwater from soaking into the ground. If you have the funds to do this, then more power to you. Just tell the contractor what to do and you are good to go. *But what if you don't have the funds to do this?*

Well, unless you are handy with a trowel, having concrete poured around the outside of your home might be outside of your budget. I know what you are thinking because I had the same thought, is there a less expensive option?

As a matter of fact, there is. You can line the area with a protective membrane for less than $100. This will run around the entire perimeter of an average-sized home. This is a DIY project most homeowners can do over a weekend. It's simple, effective, and it's as cheap as chips. No backup pumps, no expensive French drain, and no butt-crack showing contractors digging up your nice new lawn.

When it's done right, installing a waterproof barrier will deflect rainwater away from your home. Seriously, it works like a charm. I've done it more times than I can shake a hairy stick at and it's never let me down.

Here's how you do it in ten easy steps.

1: Pick up a roll of thick, black plastic from the hardware store.

2: Remove any flowerbeds, bushes, etc. from the perimeter of your foundation.

3: Grade the soil away from your foundation using a rake. Depending on the lay of the land, you may need to remove some soil or bring some in some extra soil/sand.

4: Roll out the plastic making sure that there's nothing sharp under it like a twig poking up. This could puncture the thick plastic and allow water to seep in.

5: Any joins must overlap by at least 4ft so that no water can work its way in.

6: Allow the plastic to run up the wall of the foundation and hold it in place with a tack to prevent it from falling.

7: Ideally, let the plastic cover run 10 ft. or more around the perimeter of your foundation.

8: Once the plastic is in place, have a load of decorative gravel delivered to your home. If you aren't sure how much to buy, show the delivery company a photo of the area, they'll estimate it for you.

9: Use a wheelbarrow to slowly tip gravel onto the plastic. Grade the gravel away from the property with a rake.

10: Once the gravel is finished, trim off any excess plastic that's sticking out.

If any of this is beyond your skill set, simply hire a local handyman and show him this image

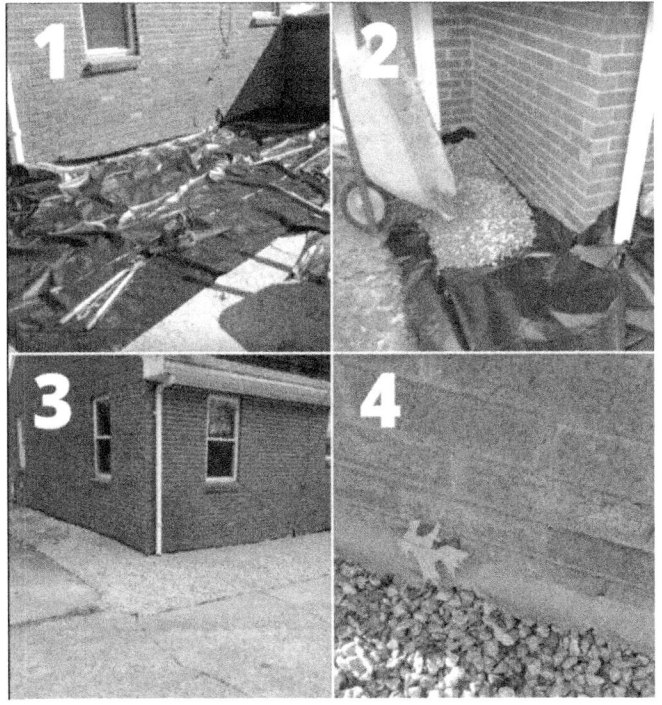

At all times, make sure that the ground slopes *away* from your property.

As a side note: If you opt for decorative gravel then don't waste your money buying it in bags. They don't go very far and it'll soon get expensive. Instead, have your local landscaping company deliver it. On average, a yard of gravel costs around $65. As a rule of thumb, a small house will take approx. three yards.

Once all of the black plastic is covered over, you can seal the edge with a neat line of mortar. Don't be put off by this final step, it's as easy as icing a cake. For any gardeners, you can soften the look of the area with plant pots. Obviously, digging holes in the plastic for flowers would be counterproductive.

BELOW GROUND WINDOWS

Basement windows are another area prone to leaks. Anytime a window is set below ground level it's as helpful as putting windows on a submarine. Sooner or later, they *will* leak.

Over the years, I've seen all kinds of fancy contraptions to try and keep out the rain and snow but sadly, none of them work. In this case, your best option is also the least expensive. Simply brick the window up. Preferably do this before you run the black, plastic sheeting. Water will now run away from your foundation.

As a final note, be sure to use the thick, black plastic sold in most hardware stores. Using a thin grade plastic won't stand up to the test of time. Hope it helps

Chapter 9: Outdoor checklist

There's an old expression - chase three chickens, catch none. This implies that problems are best tackled one at a time. Earlier, we learned that mold needs three things to thrive, a food source, humidity, and water. In this chapter, we'll focus on a few more ways that water can work its way into your home. Let's start at the top and work our way down.

Rooflines come in all shapes and sizes. The more complicated the roof, the higher the probability of water finding its way in. Flat roofs and roofs with built-in skylights are particularly prone to leaks. This is something to keep in mind when buying a new home. Obviously, this applies to renters too.

Anything that pokes out of your roof like a vent pipe, a chimney stack, or a dormer window, is worthy of an inspection. You can do this from the safety of the sidewalk with the help of an inexpensive pair of binoculars. This also allows you to scour the roofline for missing roof shingles. Missing roof shingles are a sure way for rainwater to find a way into your attic space.

Gutters and downspouts are there to direct rainwater away from your home. During a rainstorm, you may have noticed how water gushes out at the bottom. Ideally, this water should drain away freely from your property. If it forms a puddle, try adding a flexible extension to the downspout. If you are using the gravel method described in the previous chapter, an easy fix is to ask your handyman/contractor/wife to mix some mortar and have them use it to direct rainwater away from the bottom of the downspout as in the following image.

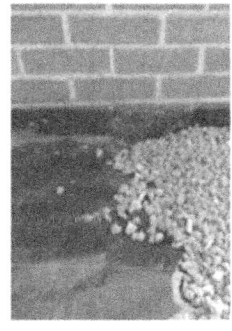 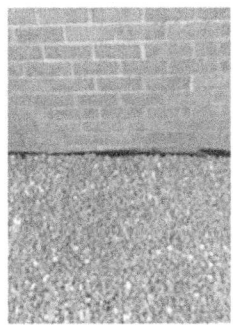 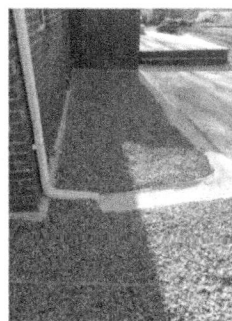

This is a simple, inexpensive way to keep all that rainwater well away from your foundation.

Do your gutters have a habit of becoming blocked with leaves? If so, it's worth installing leaf guards. Leaf guards are effective at what they do. Failing that, grab yourself a ladder and make gutter cleaning a part of your fall cleanup routine. To help you understand why rainwater needs to move away from your home, imagine a house at the top of a hill with torrential rain bouncing off the roof. *Can you see it?*

As the rain gushes out of the downspout, it will begin to run down the hill. This is good news for the homeowner but not so good for his imaginary neighbor living at the bottom of the hill. No matter how hard this poor fella tries, his battle with groundwater is reliant on other people. (Something else to keep in mind when shopping for a new home).

Sadly, you don't have to live at the bottom of a hill to inherit someone else's rainwater. Nope, even a slight variation in the land can send gallons of unwanted rainwater to your property. Water always seems to find the path of least resistance.

Whenever I see homeowners battling with groundwater, it's usually because they can't see the wood for the trees. Tall garden fences, hedges, and other buildings can obscure a person's perception. It isn't until I ask homeowners to take a few steps back that they have a more accurate appreciation for the lay of the land.

Look, we all know that a new home is an emotional purchase. That white picket fence always looks so pretty in the mid-afternoon sun. But before you sign anything, I would urge you to stand across the road and ask yourself, where is your neighbor's rainwater going to settle?

In water-damaged homes, water is easy to suck up. Before you know it, that water damaged home looks like any other. But was the flooded area treated for mold? If not, you could be moving into a home with a hidden problem. With that in mind, it would be prudent to go and knock on a few doors and ask if the street has flooded in the past. History *always* repeats itself.

Now that I have that tip out of the way, let's press on and see if there are any other potential problems you might not be aware of.

LAWN AND GARDEN

If I had a dollar for every sprinkler I'd seen soaking the side of a house I wouldn't be writing any more books. Instead, I'd be sitting on a white sandy beach smoking a Cuban cigar. Seriously, I've seen my fair share of misplaced sprinklers.

Sprinklers placed too close to a building can cause damp. Depending on how long it has been running, damp can penetrate the outer wall. To add to the problem, all that water is again trickling down to the foundation. Thankfully, this problem is a really easy one fix, just move the darn sprinkler. While you are at it, feel free to check that any flowerbeds, garden soil, or mulch all slope away from the foundation. This will also help to keep rainwater moving away from the area.

GARAGE AND CAR

Anything you store in the garage such as fishing or camping equipment should be put away dry. This brings us to the ominous topic of flood-damaged vehicles.

Believe it or not, there's an entire market dedicated to buying and selling flood-damaged cars. Once a car has been totaled, dealers can buy them from insurance companies at knock-down prices. There are thousands of these cars circulating. In most cases, buyers have no idea that the car they are driving has been underwater. Talk about dipping your headlights, lol.

Anyways, before buying a used vehicle, always check the Carfax details. As a rule, a salvage title should show up. In some states, used car salesmen are required to make you aware of any previous defects. But as Upton Sinclair once said, "It is difficult to get a man to understand something when his salary depends upon his not understanding it."

Treat moldy cars like you would a moldy home. Don't take on big projects and be prepared to walk away from the vehicle. If you are treating smaller amounts of mold, always remember to wear a mask, gloves, and goggles.

Driving a moldy car is no different than sitting in a moldy house. If your daily commute in a new vehicle leaves you feeling more tired than usual, it pays to be diligent. Lift the carpets and feel if the underlayment is damp or smells like old socks. If so, dry the carpets out and treat the area for mold.

If your car has a sunroof, periodically check it for leaks. If you live in a place where it snows, rubber mats can help to keep the carpets dry. If you have children traveling with you, then you have fruit juice spilled on the car seats. Take the car seat out and check for signs of mold.

Leather seats and dashboards are easier to clean than soft fabrics. These types of hard surfaces can be cleaned with white vinegar or ammonia. To use ammonia simply mix it 50/50 with water and apply it to the area with a spray bottle. You might want to open the windows while you do this.

Let the ammonia sit for an hour or two and wipe the area down with a damp cloth. As a side note, *never* combine ammonia with bleach or chlorine. It will produce poisonous gases.

Distilled vinegar is a much gentler option. White vinegar is effective at killing roughly 82% of mold species. If you have small children and pets, this is a better option than using ammonia or bleach.

To use, simply pour the vinegar into a spray bottle and spray it onto the mold. After letting it sit for an hour, wipe it down with a damp cloth, then dry.

Fabric seats are best treated with an antimicrobial solution. Allow to dry and vacuum the seats with a HEPA vax.

Most people forget this but vehicles are fitted with their own cabin filter. They are designed to filter out fine dust particles. This helps to keep the air in your vehicle clean whenever you turn the heat/AC on. Once you have located your vehicle's cabin filter, they are easy to super easy to replace. Cabin filters should be replaced once a year, or every 10,000 miles, whichever comes first.

Chapter 10: Indoor checklist

Fixing leaks and dealing with poor ventilation are the keys to controlling mold. Straight out of the gate, let's head up to the attic and see if there is anything amiss up there.

Attics tend to get hot in the summer and cold in winter. The two things controlling excess moisture are ventilation and insulation.

Open your attic door and you should be able to see a layer of insulation laid on the floor. The space between this insulation and the rest of the roof space needs to be vented.

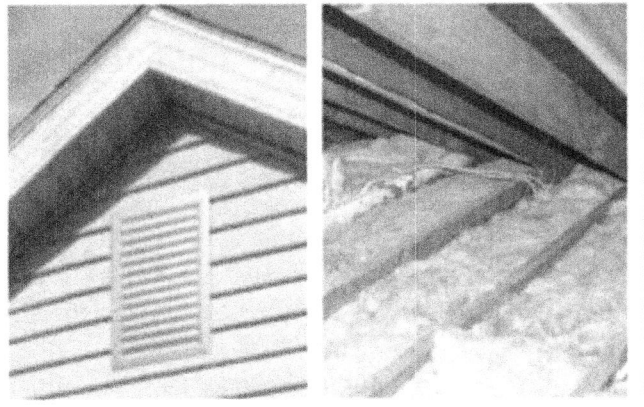

In hot climates, many homeowners skip insulation thinking its only purpose is to keep the heat in. But that's not the case. A properly insulated attic can also help keep a house cool in summer. This, in turn, will help to lower energy bills.

In cold climates, a layer of insulation prevents heat from escaping through the roof. But this time around, it's not just about saving energy. If warm air was allowed to meet a snow-covered roof, then ice dams would form on the outside of the roof. *That's not good right?*

Not unless you want an attic full of ice. Ice dams can easily work their way under roofing shingles. Once the ice melts, it creates excess moisture and it becomes a perfect growing environment for mold. For this reason, it's best to keep attics as cool as the outside temperatures. In the construction trade, this is sometimes described as "keeping a cold roof."

Roof vents help with this as they allow outside air to circulate freely through the attic. To comply with building codes newer homes may have the vents built into the roof. Whereas older homes usually have louvered vents situated on each end of the house. It really doesn't matter which type you have, so long as air circulates freely. When inspecting your attic, make sure these vents aren't obstructed in any way, shape, or form.

Also, check your attic for signs of a leaking roof. A flashlight comes in handy for those dark corners. If you have a chimney running up through the attic, pay close attention to any wet brickwork. Chimneys are sealed to the roof with lead flashing. If it's not installed properly, it can be prone to leaks. If any leaks are detected, get them fixed quickly. Procrastination is a friend of mold!

Working our way down out of the attic, now pay close attention to your bedroom ceilings. Watermarks can offer a valuable clue to a less obvious roof leak. Plumbing leaks can be a little harder to detect as they can hide inside wall cavities. But all is not lost.

Allergy flare-ups are a good indicator that mold is hiding inside a wall. Remember, some molds will have a distinct musty, earthy smell. Others can resemble wet socks or even cat urine!

As you look around your home, be sure to keep a sharp eye on any wall that joins a bathroom or kitchen. Peeling wallpaper should be an instant red flag, especially if it has been painted over. This seals in the moisture and creates another fine environment for mold to grow in.

BEDROOMS

Most people enjoy the feeling of a soft carpet when stepping out of bed. Not me. I know that wall to wall carpet can be a magnet for mold. Solid wood floors tend to fare much better, as do tiled floors. But that doesn't mean you have to go without your creature comforts. A removable area rug will add a touch of style. It's also easier to pick up and clean after an accidental spill.

While checking the bedroom, look inside stuffy bedroom closets and behind large pieces of bedroom furniture. Both can stifle airflow and encourage mold to grow. Anytime you stumble across a mold type substance, treat it as superman would kryptonite. Gloves, goggles, and a respirator are your best protection from toxic mold.

House plants add a nice touch to any room. They can also help to improve indoor air quality. The trick is not to overwater them. Plants sitting in a puddle of water are an ideal way to help any mold spores grow.

BATHROOMS

Any room with running water has the potential to cause a problem. Bathrooms are a firm favorite for mold as hot showers generate lots of excess moisture. The key to preventing this is to install a fan that's powerful enough to match the level of the stream being created. A bathroom with an ineffective fan is about as much use as an ashtray on a motorcycle.

To discourage mold from growing, humidity is best kept between 30% and 50%. An inexpensive humidity meter hanging on the bathroom wall can help to keep a track of this.

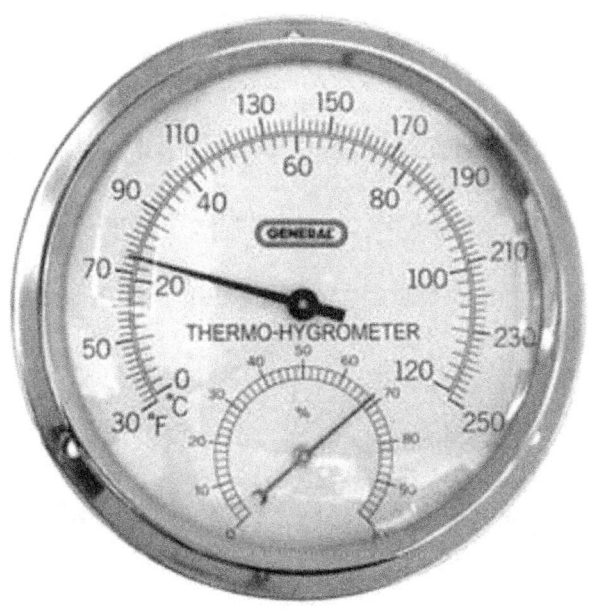

As an added bonus, low humidity also discourages cockroaches and dust mites. If you are on a tight budget, and your bathroom doesn't have a fan, always open the window when taking a shower. Whenever you finish using the shower, it's a good habit to remove any damp towels from the bathroom. All too often, they sit in the bottom of a damp, wicker laundry basket. Bathmats, sponges, and wash clothes should also be changed out regularly.

Check the grout between bathroom tiles. Unless it's been sealed, the grout is porous which is why mold likes to grow there. If you are just discovering this after the tiles have been installed, all is not lost. Hardware stores sell a spray-on sealer. Once the mold has been removed, spray the sealer onto the grout. This works like a charm and will stop mold from growing back.

Shower liners with a hem at the bottom tend to hold water. This is a sneaky one so replace shower liners often before they become a mini mold trap. Fortunately, new shower liners are pretty cheap to buy.

Before we leave the bathroom, check for obvious signs of leaks under the bathroom sink and around the toilet area. A small drip over a long period can easily lead to a big mold issue.

KITCHEN

More leaks occur under the kitchen sink than in any other place in the home. Oftentimes, water can seep into the surrounding cupboard. Again, a flashlight can help pinpoint leaks. While you have your head under the sink check that it is sealed to the countertop. During installation, some plumbers miss this step and water gets into the countertop. Catching it early can save you hundreds of dollars in replaced counters.

Damp sponges left on countertops should be rotated often. Simply toss them in your washing machine along with any dish towels. Adding a cup of borax to the wash will help kill any mold spores. If they are pretty nasty, you can also let them soak overnight in a bucket of water mixed with 1 cup ammonia and half a cup of borax.

While we are in the kitchen, let us not forget that mold can be ingested. Yup, it's true, people inadvertently eat mold all the time. If you have family, I'd bet the farm something is sitting at the back of your fridge right now that's out of date or moldy.

For people with a healthy immune system, eating a small amount of mold isn't likely to kill you. Although it could induce nausea and vomiting. A good way to avoid this is to have a date set on your phone to clean the fridge out.

MOPS

Kitchen mops get a bit of a raw deal in this life. We use them to wipe over our dirty floors and then put them away in a dark closet, usually cold and wet. In a confined space, this is a breeding ground for bacteria and mold. A much better option is to wash the mop out and then store it upside down, preferably outside. Direct sunlight will help to disinfect the mop. *No really, it's true.*

VENTS

Cooking smells are best vented out of the kitchen. The vent should be directed to an outside wall. This will prevent warm, humid air from escaping into wall cavities. Believe it or not, I once saw a stovetop vented directly into the basement. Needless to say, it was the primary cause of toxic mold.

With that in mind, it wouldn't hurt to check where your stovetop vent leads to. Simply turn on the fan and look for signs of air moving through any visible vents. If you can't see any, it could be a potential problem. Fortunately, running new ductwork isn't likely to break the bank.

MERRY MOLD

I know we covered basement issues earlier but it's worth repeating. If your goal is to live in a house free of toxic mold, then you might want to rethink what you bring up from the basement. As hard as it is, it's best to toss that moldy old Christmas tree and start again. Feel free to pause here and ask yourself, "how much is your health worth to you?"

Chapter 11: Mold big guns

Finding and treating excess moisture in your home is paramount to the success of your mold remediation project. Put simply, if you ain't fixed the leaks, you ain't gonna fix the mold.

Also keep in mind, that the goal of remediation isn't to kill mold, it's to remove it. Dead or weakened mold spores left lying around on the floor still pose a health risk. Think of mold remediation like killing flies with fly spray. Some of the flies will die, others might continue to wiggle around a bit. Either way, you wouldn't want to leave them on your kitchen floor.

Now that we have that little analogy out of the way, we'll look at some of the tools used in mold remediation. If money is too tight to mention, then you should be able to find each of these items at your local rental store.

FOGGERS:

A mold fogger is a device that can turn any liquid mold solution (such as a fungicide) into a fine mist/fog, hence the name. I know what you are thinking because I had the same thought. Why would anyone want to spend good money turning a liquid into a fog when you could put it in a spray bottle?

Well, foggers do a fantastic job of distributing mold solutions over a large area. They do this evenly which helps to cut down on waste. But the main advantage of foggers is that they can get into those hard to reach areas. When it comes to small cracks and crevices, foggers are the real deal.

By the time you notice mold growing on a wall, it can be the tip of the iceberg. Those microscopic, mold spores can be present throughout an entire room. Foggers help to saturate the area while getting to those spores that are invisible to the naked eye.

AIR SCRUBBERS

An air scrubber is a portable filtration system. It's designed to remove fine particles from the air. It does this by sucking in air from the environment and then passes it through a series of filters. This, in turn, helps to improve indoor air quality.

Air scrubbers can be fitted with different filters to meet different hazards. The type of filter used to remove mold spores is our old friend the HEPA filter.

Air scrubbers improve air quality quickly. They operate on the principle of negative airflow. As we learned earlier, negative airflow simply means it removes air in a room faster than it is replaced. This makes a cleaner, safer environment for people to work in.

Air scrubbers come in a variety of sizes and you'll need to get one to match your needs. Air scrubbers also have two air cleaning options, dry scrubbing, and wet scrubbing. Wet scrubbing traps contaminants by sucking air through a damp pad or filter. Dry scrubbing sucks contaminants through a dry filter.

Air scrubbers are mostly used in commercial settings. Although, some air scrubbers fit into HVAC systems (Heating, Ventilation, and Air Conditioning). As air passes through the ductwork, it is then scrubbed and purified.

Before using a rented air scrubber, always check the filters and seals for signs of wear and tear. Air scrubbers cannot work properly if the air is escaping, or if the filters are blocked. You can request a new filter at the time of renting.

DEHUMIDIFIER

Dehumidifiers are designed to pull excess moisture out of the air. They don't kill mold, but they do prevent it by reducing humidity. Humidity is measured by the amount of water vapor in the air. Any place with excess moisture will help mold to grow.

A small dehumidifier can absorb up to thirty pints of water per day. Larger ones up to ninety pints per day. They do this by drawing moist air into the dehumidifier which then crosses over a set of cool coils. As it does so, moisture is condensed.

High powered fans and air movers are okay at a pinch. Obviously, you'll want them pointing directly outside to reduce the number of mold spores blowing around. If you don't have access to an open door or window you might want to give blowers a miss.

HEPA VACUUM

Following mold remediation (such as "fogging)," mold spores and mycotoxins become heavy and fall to the ground. Left to their own devices, they have the potential to become a source of toxicity. Yup, that old chestnut, so it's not enough to just kill the mold, dead spores must also be removed.

A regular vacuum cleaner isn't going to cut it. Mold spores and mycotoxins are far too small and they will pass right through the filter.

HEPA vacuum cleaners work on the same principle as a regular vacuum cleaner. What sets it apart is the filter. HEPA filters capture particles smaller than 0.3 microns. Even this isn't small enough to catch every single mold spore and mycotoxin in your home. The best we can hope for is to remove 99.97% of them. The tiny fraction that remains can be managed with the practices mentioned in this book.

As a side note: Early use of HEPA filters dates back to the Second World War. They were designed to capture radioactive particles released by the atomic bomb! Today, they are more popular with people who work in the mold industry.

Chapter 12: Hire a pro without getting ripped off

Dealing with a mold outbreak is frustrating at the best of times. So, when a company offers to do a free mold inspection, it can seem like you are finally catching a break.

Let's be clear, "free" is a tactic used by some in the mold industry to get a foot in the door. As I've said before, when it comes to mold remediation, ain't nothing for nothing.

Anytime you see the word "free" ask yourself, why would an honest person, let alone a stranger want to work for free? The truth is, whenever something sounds too good to be true, it probably is. So, if you see an advertisement offering a free mold test or a free mold inspection, it's a scam.

People who operate this way are looking for a way to drum up business. Unfortunately, they have a nasty habit of finding it. Simple mold jobs like a new water stain become an over-exaggerated Mold-ageddon type problem that only they can fix.

To put this into context, the vast majority of mold inspectors are decent, honest people. As such, honest people are in high demand which makes them less inclined to push free services. Why would they?

That said, if you have a mold problem, **find a mold inspector that has zero interest in doing the mold remediation work.** This takes away any potential conflict of interest. Ideally, choose a local inspector and ask for references.

When you hire someone locally, it also makes any callbacks easier to deal with. The same applies to mold remediation companies. A small, local businessman will usually work harder to keep you happy. It's the local aspect that makes people more accountable. Nobody wants to bump into an unhappy customer at the grocery store who feels like they were ripped off.

Hiring someone local also makes checking those references easier. They might even be people in your town who you know. Keep this in mind when you see mold companies advertising on national TV.

With thousands of dollars at stake, fraud and deception can happen in any industry. I'm just asking you to be vigilant. Always, always, always ask for a written estimate and have them break down the cost of the work to be carried out. Ideally, get three estimates and then compare them.

Any person that can't break down an estimate, or appears pushy on the phone, should be an instant red flag.

Once the mold remediation company has finished, they will be keen to get paid for the work. There is nothing wrong with being keen or getting paid for a job well done, but the area should be re-tested for mold. This is where that unbiased mold inspector comes in handy.

A post-remediation test should always be done by a third party. Follow these simple steps and you will have peace of mind that the job is done right, and you won't have to overpay in the process. Don't hand over your hard-earned money until you have a document in your hand verifying that the mold remediation was successful. If you have to, tell them I said so.

Chapter 13: Covered Ground

We seem to have covered a lot of ground in a short time. Hopefully, you have learned something new and perhaps even smiled somewhere along the way. I try to use a little humor when I write as it makes the topics more interesting.

Before we close, let's quickly recap.

Mold spores are all around us. They like to grow in places where moisture is elevated and ventilation is poor. They feed on porous materials and any porous material will do. Mold is particularly fond of basement clutter and drywall. This makes water-damaged buildings, attics, basements, bathrooms, and kitchens all willing candidates.

Testing your home for mold can be helpful. Although nobody knows for sure how many different mold species there are. **What you don't want to find is dangerous molds circulating at high levels.**

Once the mold gets established, it can cause a wide range of health problems. Most doctors who practice mainstream medicine are blissfully unaware of mold-related illnesses.

The fastest, most efficient way to separate yourself from toxic mold is to run like hell. Find a cleaner home and start over. Owning fewer possessions will make this transition easier.

While searching for a new home, pay close attention to the ground the property is built on. Ideally, find a place where rainwater drains away freely. Don't be afraid to knock on a few doors and ask any would-be neighbors if the street has flooded in the past.

For those who stay and fight mold, a local mold inspector is a good person to have on your team. But avoid using anyone that might have a conflict of interest. If a mold remediation bill is more than a thousand dollars, ask for an itemized estimate. Then cross-check the numbers by getting two more estimates.

When tackling small mold projects, it's important to protect yourself with mold rated PPE. Even then, small outbreaks of mold are best tackled by those in good health.

Cross-contamination of mold spores can happen at lightning speed. Be sure to isolate any rooms with plastic sheeting. A fan in the window blowing outwards will also help to send any airborne spores outside.

Use the indoor and outdoor checklist in this book to help locate potential problems. If you find one, spraying bleach on mold can make matters worse. An antimicrobial will render much better results.

Attics need ventilation and remember that simple roofs are less prone to leaks. Any leaks should be dealt with quickly. A dehumidifier can help to dry areas out.

Foggers, Air scrubbers, and HEPA vacuums can all help you deal with mold. However, **your best ally is a robust immune system.** You can learn how to optimize your immune system in my first book titled, *The Healing Point*.

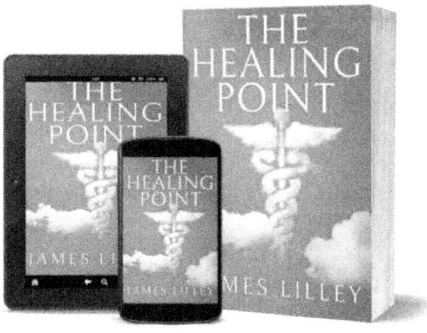

For now, I guess that's it except to say thank *you* for spending your valuable time with me. I hope you found this information helpful. If so, could I trouble you for a short review? **It doesn't have to be anything fancy, a simple sentence will do.** As a small, independent author I rely on word of mouth for every book sale.

Last but not least, thank you to my wife and family. Without their support, writing these books would not be possible.

Until next time, bye for now,

James.

More books by this author

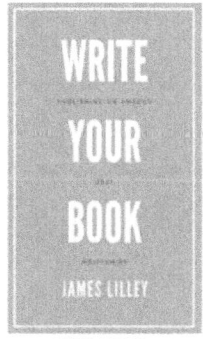 HOW TO

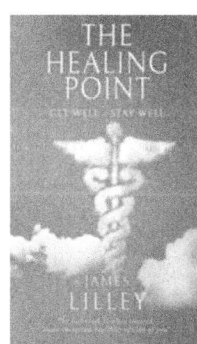 IMMUNE BOOST

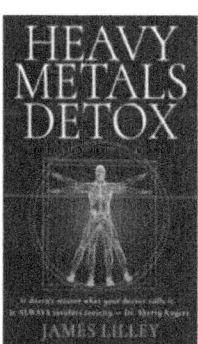 DETOXIFICATION

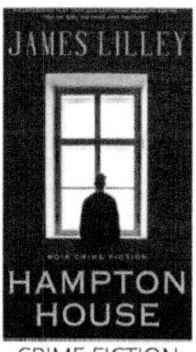 CRIME FICTION

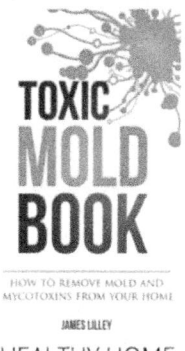 HEALTHY HOME

MORE SOON!

I'm currently working on a new fiction book. If you would like a chance to see **your name** in print be sure to stay in my loop at *writeonjames.com*. I sometimes run fun competitions where the winning names become the main characters! The newsletter will also let you know when I have a new book coming out.

Newsletter

WriteonJames.com

Thank you for your support, I genuinely appreciate it.

James.

NOTES

NOTES

NOTES

Printed in Dunstable, United Kingdom